GLUTEN-FREE SOURDOUGH COOKBOOK

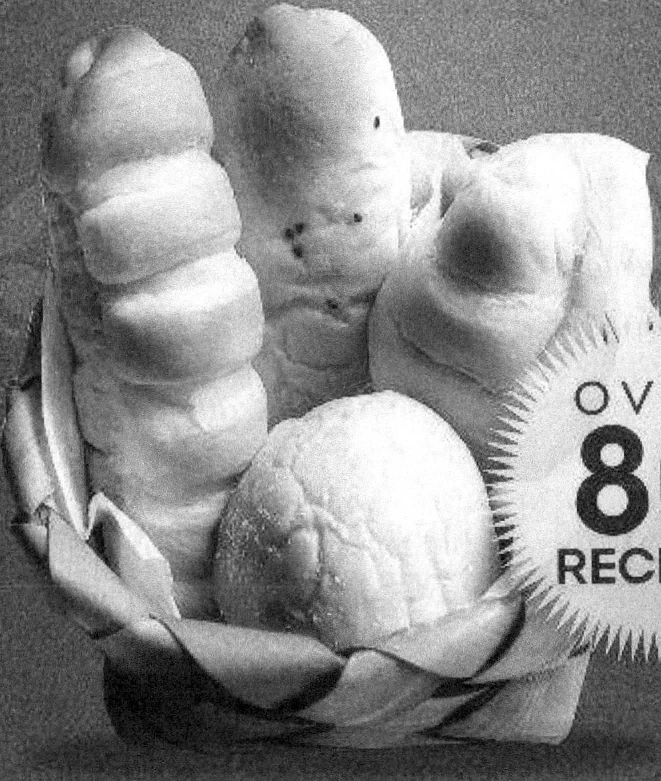

OVER 80 RECIPES

KIMBERLY WRIGHT

COPYRIGHT

Dear Beautiful Souls,

Your thoughts and views are priceless treasures in our quest to create content that resonates with you. If this book brought you a smile or peace, we urge you to express your thoughts through a passionate review. Your input is a priceless gift that allows us to improve our materials and make them even more pleasurable for other Sourdough fanatics and enthusiasts alike.

In gratitude for your kindness,

TABLE OF CONTENTS

Do you recall when "gluten-free bread" was just a depressing cardboard replica of the real thing? Yes, I supposed. But, my sourdough-curious and gluten-free fighters, those days are definitely gone! Hang in tight because we're about to set out on a delectable journey into a universe devoid of any gluten, filled with fluffy clouds of crumb, explosive flavour, and crusty joy!

This cookbook isn't some enchanted Pinterest board with ambiguous guidelines. I'm Kimberly Wright, a self-taught alchemist of sourdough who has had many baking victories as well as scorched loaves. Even if your kitchen is more like a little studio apartment, I'm here to offer the tips, techniques and sourdough zen that will turn you from beginner to expert and give you the confidence of a Parisian chef while baking.

Now let's talk about the big problem in the room: the bread. Put cardboard aside. We're talking about rustic sourdough loaves with a crumb so light it almost floats and that crackle like a crackling fire. Imagine biting into a crisp, thin pizza crust that matches that of Naples or sinking your teeth into a zesty focaccia filled with fresh herbs and olive oil. Yes, there are sweet goodies available as well, such as banana bread and cinnamon buns, which are so fluffy and full of flavour that they could make angels weep.

Let's first discuss your sourdough starter, which is the foundation of our adventure, before getting started with the dough. This small habitat of bubbling microorganisms is going to be your baking spirit animal and closest buddy. We'll take care of feeding schedules expertly, explain the workings of fermentation, and address any odd smells that may surface (believe me, we've all been there!).

When baking gluten-free seemed like a guessing game, do you recall those days? Not anymore! We'll unravel the mysteries behind gluten-free flour mixes, interpreting their characteristics and discovering how to mix them like a seasoned alchemist. No matter the size of your kitchen, you'll be producing crispy baguettes and fluffy focaccia with the assurance of an experienced baker.

Not to be overlooked is the sweet aspect of sourdough. We'll create sourdough waffles that are light, fluffy, and full of tangy taste, as well as cinnamon buns that would make your grandmother envy and banana bread so moist you'll have to doubt reality.

This is a journey about empowerment, not simply baking. It's about rediscovering the delight of freshly baked bread, the fulfilment that comes from making something enchanted from scratch, and the self-assurance to serve it to those you love. Now throw away the store-bought ingredients, take out your whisk, and let's start fermenting!

This cookbook is a roadmap to a world of delectable possibilities, not simply a guide. All you gluten-free bakers out there, are you prepared to shine? Come on, let's bake!

CHAPTER 1

"Gluten-free baking" may make the uninformed picture thick, cardboard blocks masquerading as bread. But do not be alarmed, daring baker! The world of gluten-free cooking has wholly changed, going from a frustrating place to a thriving one full of culinary opportunities. Today's world of gluten-free baking is an exciting playground where you may discover flavours, textures, and sensations you never knew existed. Forget about tasteless flours and gummy textures.

The era of substituting only one flour is over. Our colour pallet has grown to encompass a symphony of options. The earthy depth of buckwheat and the light and delicate almond flour combine, while the rich sweetness of sorghum provides structure to the whole affair. Hazelnut flour's mild nuttiness lends a hint of elegance, while coconut flour, a scene-stealer due to its absorbent nature, works wonders to produce airy marvels. Every flour has its unique personality, abilities, and eccentricities that are just waiting to be explored and grasped.

But half the joy is in getting to know these characters. The artistry starts with learning how they interact and how they dance in the mixing bowl. Combining several flours creates a rainbow of tastes and sensations. Brown rice and sorghum combine to make crusty loaves with a pleasing crunch, and almonds and coconut combine to make delicate cakes. You follow your experiments, and every dish is a delectable journey through the magic of flour.

And then there's the hydration magic. The seemingly straightforward molecule of water acts as the director of your baking symphony. A little more may turn a thick brick into a fluffy cloud, while a little less can result in a golden crust that cracks. Acquiring the skill to tune in to your dough and sense its minute alterations transforms into a personal dance of touch and understanding.

The Tangy Symphony of Fermentation: The Enchantment of Sourdough Science

The age-old dance of bacteria known as fermentation is becoming more than just a catchphrase in gluten-free baking. It's the undiscovered tool that turns your works of art from excellent to extraordinary. In addition to leavening your bread, these microscopic yeasts and bacteria that are chowing down on sugars also release a symphony of flavours that would make dull wheat loaves cry with jealousy.

The gifts of fermentation include the delicate nutty flavour of whole grains, the touch of sweetness from caramelized sugars, and the tangy kiss of lactic acid. Their intricate weaving leaves your taste senses yearning for more. And how lovely is sourdough? It's a co-creative, living ecosystem that you tend to as your little culinary pet.

Feeding your starter, watching it burst into life, and then experiencing its transforming power in your baked goods is a beautiful and satisfying experience. As you weave flavour and texture from the most essential components, you become a collaborator in creation and a conductor of microbial magic.

Crafting Your Starter: Flourishing From Scratch

However, how might this masterwork of microbes be unlocked? Making your sourdough starter is an exciting experience filled with expectation and learning. Selecting flour, providing your nascent colony with cautious sustenance, and observing its initial victorious ascent are experiences that every gluten-free baker must share.

In creating your starter, there is no one "right" way to do it. While some believe rye to be a more receptive muse, others swear to organic whole wheat. While some bakers swear on the power of silent contemplation, others serenade their starter with jazz music. But one thing always stays the same: the secret is patience.

Don't let a sluggish starter or several seemingly inactivity days deter you. Your microbe pals are just getting used to their new surroundings and picking up the rhythm of your kitchen. They'll soon thank you with their vibrant excitement and be ready to bring your gluten-free baking to life with loving care and regular feedings.

Thus, inhale deeply, muster your courage, and venture into the fascinating realm of gluten-free baking. You may soon be creating loaves that are on par with everything the wheat world has to offer if you have an open mind, a keen palate, and a willingness to try new things. The tricks of your craft, the keys to unlocking gluten-free heaven, are the combinations of wheat, the dance of hydration, and the enchantment of fermentation. Go ahead and bake now!

Sourdough Varieties

CHAPTER 2

Cultivating Your Sourdough Soul mate

In the realm of gluten-free baking, sourdough is more than just a leavening agent; it's a living companion, a vibrant sourdough starter bubbling with life and potential. However, maintaining this microbial muse requires some care, much like any relationship. Gather your whisk and get ready to go on an enlightening voyage where we will help you make your very own sourdough soul mate, solve everyday problems, and reveal the secrets of a thriving starter that will support your baking endeavours for years to come.

The Life's Spark: Crafting Your Starter

Your sourdough starter doesn't require a kiss to awaken, so throw away the fairy tales. A basic mixture of flour and water, a little perseverance, and a dash of curiosity are all that are needed. A typical option is organic whole wheat flour, which is a home for a variety of bacteria. However, you can also find inspiration with rye, spelt, or even a gluten-free combination like brown rice and sorghum. Recall that each flour gives your starter a distinct personality that affects its rise and flavour profile, just like fingerprints do.

Now, make a thick batter by combining your preferred flour with warm water. Consider it your little pals, the bacteria and yeast, having a comfortable apartment Cover it loosely and tuck it away in a warm, dark corner – your kitchen counter or a cozy oven with the light turned off will do the trick. Your starter won't miraculously come to life overnight, so patience is essential. But after a day or two, you'll see the first indications of life: little bubbles bursting through the surface and a faint smell of yeast in the air. This marks the start of your incredible connection and the spark of life.

Nurturing the Flame – Feeding Schedules and Storage Tips

Just like any relationship, your starter needs regular TLC to thrive. Give your starter a "meal" of fresh flour and water once every 12 to 24 hours, depending on the flour you use and its ambient temperature. Remove half of the combination that is already there (we'll refer to this as your "discard"—your culinary treasure, but more on that later!), then swap it out for an equal amount of new flour and water. Gently stir while observing the dough come to life and the bubbles dancing.

Maintaining consistency is essential. Think of it like a regular date night for your starter. Even if feedings are only done once a day, follow a strict schedule. If you don't witness regular activity right away, don't panic; some starters need a week or two to awaken completely. All you need to do is keep feeding and observing, and before long, you'll have a lively, effervescent friend who is ready to bake with.

But where does your starter live when it's not baking? Its ideal refuge is a plain glass jar or ceramic container. Steer clear of metal as it might change the pH and impede fermentation. Store your starter at room temperature, preferably away from direct sunlight and drafts. A warm starter makes a happy starter, so if your kitchen is too cold, think about finding a warm area next to an oven or heater (that should be switched off, of course!).

Troubleshooting Woes – Conquering Slow Rise, Inactivity, and Funky Smells

Even the best relationships face challenges. If your starting appears slow or acts a little out of control with strange scents, don't worry. These are only hiccups on the path to baking happiness, and you can quickly get back on course with a bit of understanding.

Slow rise? Give a slight boost to your Starter. Sometimes, it comes back to life with a warm water bath or a peek inside the oven with the light on. Try using a different flour if, after a week, your Starter still doesn't seem to be active. While some starters love the sweetness of brown rice, others like the stronger flavour of rye. Play around and discover what kindles the flame in your Starter.

Funky smells? Remain calm! While a slight yeasty scent is Okay, acetone or vinegar odours in your Starter may indicate carelessness. Boost the number of times you feed it, toss out more of the previous mixture, and stir it well. To combat unpleasant odours, keep in mind that fresh ingredients and a clean container are your best allies.

With a bit of perseverance, understanding, and curiosity, you may quickly have a healthy sourdough starter that serves as more than simply a leavening agent—instead, it becomes your reliable baking companion, your culinary confidante, and the key to opening up a world of delectable gluten-free recipes. Now go forth and bake, and always remember that the journey is worth as much as the outcome!

CHAPTER 3

Mediterranean Sunburst Sourdough

Yield: 1 large loaf, about 10 slices

Prep: 15 mins, Rise: 4-6 hours, baking: 45 mins

Ingredients:

Equal parts brown rice and millet flour (1 ½ cups each)

Yeast (1 teaspoon)

Salt (1 ½ teaspoons)

Honey (1 tablespoon)

Warm water (1 ¼ cup, pleasantly warm)

Sun-dried tomatoes, chopped (½ cup)

Kalamata olives, chopped (¼ cup)

Fresh basil, chopped (¼ cup)

Olive oil (2 tablespoons)

Directions:

In a spacious bowl, combine flour, yeast, and salt.

In another bowl, mix warm water and honey. Stir to form a dough with the dry ingredients. Once it has doubled in size, cover it and let it rise at room temperature for four to six hours.

Preheat the oven to 200°C or 400°F. Line a baking sheet with parchment paper.

Gently mix in the sun-dried tomatoes, olives, and basil after adding them to the dough. Transfer it to the prepared baking sheet after shaping it into a circular loaf. Pour some olive oil over it.

Bake for 45 minutes, or until the cake is golden brown and a toothpick inserted in the centre comes out clean. Before slicing, set aside on a cooling rack.

Nutrition Information:

Per slice (assuming 10 slices):

Calories: 220

Carbohydrates: 34g

Protein: 4g

Fat: 8g

Fiber: 2g

Sodium: 300mg

Caramelized Onion & Walnut Symphony Sourdough

Yield: 1 large loaf, about 10 slices

Prep: 20 mins, Rise: 4-6 hours, baking: 45 mins)

Ingredients:

Flours: 2 cups (1 spelt, 1 almond)

Dry: 1 tsp yeast, 1 ½ tsp salt

Wet: 1 tbsp honey, 1 ¼ cup warm water, 1 tbsp olive oil

Toppings: 1 large onion (thinly sliced), ½ cup walnuts (chopped), ½ tsp thyme, ¼ tsp sea salt

Directions:

In a large mixing basin, whisk together the flour, yeast, and salt.

Warm the olive oil in a spare pan at medium heat. Add the onions and simmer for approximately 15 minutes, stirring now and again, until they are caramelized and golden brown.

Add the thyme, caramelized onions, and walnuts to the dry ingredients after whisking honey into heated water. Stir to make a dough. Once it has doubled in size, cover it and let it rise at room temperature for four to six hours.

Prep oven: 400°F/200°C. Line the baking sheet with parchment.

Gently mix the remaining ¼ tsp sea salt into the dough. Transfer it to the prepared baking sheet after shaping it into a circular loaf.

Bake for 45 minutes or until golden brown, checking for doneness with a toothpick. Cool completely before slicing.

Nutrition Information:

Per slice (assuming 10 slices):

Calories: 270

Carbohydrates: 38g

Protein: 6g

Fat: 11g

Fiber: 3g

Sodium: 250mg

Smoky Gouda & Chive Surprise Sourdough

Yield: 1 large loaf, about 10 slices |

Prep: 15 mins, Rise: 4-6 hours, baking: 45 mins

Ingredients:

Starter: 1 ½ cups active sourdough starter

Flours: 1 ½ cups brown rice flour, ½ cup whole wheat flour (optional)

Seasonings: 1 tsp salt, 1 tbsp honey

Mix-ins: ¼ cup grated smoked Gouda cheese, 2 tbsp chopped fresh chives

Instructions:

Mix the flour, honey, salt, and sourdough starter in a big basin. Stir to produce a shaggy dough.

Add the chives and grated Gouda cheese and knead for five minutes. Once it has doubled in size, cover it and let it rise at room temperature for four to six hours.

Turn the oven on to 400°F or 200°C.

Line a baking sheet with parchment paper.

Very carefully, shape the dough into a round loaf. Transfer to the prepared baking sheet and score the top with a sharp knife.

Bake for 45 minutes, or until the cake is golden brown and a toothpick inserted in the centre comes out clean. Keep cool on a cooling rack before slicing.

Nutrition Information:

Per slice (assuming 10 slices):

Calories: 250

Carbohydrates: 36g

Protein: 7g

Fat: 9g

Fiber: 3g

Sodium: 350mg

Cranberry Orange Zest Celebration Sourdough

Yield: 1 large loaf, about 10 slices

Prep: 20 mins, Rise: 4-6 hours, baking: 45 mins)

Ingredients:

Flours: 2 cups (1 ½ brown rice, ½ sorghum)

Dry: 1 tsp yeast, 1 ½ tsp salt

Wet: 1 tbsp honey, 1 ¼ cup warm water

Mix-ins: 1 cup cranberries, 1 tbsp orange zest, ¼ tsp cinnamon

Directions:

In a large basin, combine flour, yeast, and salt.

Mix honey and warm water in a different dish. Incorporate cinnamon, orange zest, and cranberries into the water mixture.

Once a dough forms, pour the wet components into the dry ingredients and stir. Once risen to room temperature, cover and let rise for 4–6 hours or until doubled in size.

Ensure the oven temperature is at 400°F or 200°C. Cover one-half of a baking sheet with parchment paper.

Gently fold in the dough to distribute the orange zest and cranberries properly. Place onto the baking sheet that has been preheated, then form into a circular loaf.

Bake for forty-five minutes, or until the top is golden brown and a toothpick inserted in the centre comes out clean. Before slicing, allow it to cool on a wire rack.

Nutrition Information:

Per slice (assuming 10 slices):

Calories: 230

Carbohydrates: 33g

Protein: 3g

Fat: 5g

Fiber: 4g

Sodium: 220mg

Rosemary & Garlic Tuscan Twist

Yield: 12 rolls

Prep: 20 mins, Rise: 2-3 hours, baking: 20 mins)

Ingredients:

Sourdough starter: 1 cup

Flour: 1 cup (all-purpose or gluten-free blend)

Salt: ½ tsp

Olive oil: 2 tbsp

Rosemary: 1-2 tsp chopped (fresh)

Garlic: 1-2 cloves minced (optional)

Directions:

Sourdough starter, flour, salt, olive oil, and rosemary should all be combined in a big basin.

Stir to produce a shaggy dough. Work the dough on a lightly floured surface for 5-10 minutes, aiming for a smooth and elastic texture.

After the dough has been oiled and covered with a wet towel, let it rise in a warm location for two to three hours or until it has doubled in size.

Make sure the oven is set to 190°C or 375°F. Line a baking sheet with parchment paper.

After deflating the dough somewhat, roll it out into a about 12-by-8-inch rectangle on a surface dusted with flour.

Cover the dough surface with the remaining 1-2 tablespoons of olive oil. Add more rosemary and minced garlic, if preferred.

Beginning with the long side, tightly roll the dough. To seal, pinch the ends shut. Divide the roll of dough into 12 equal pieces.

Leave room between each roll so that they may rise, and arrange the rolls on the prepared baking sheet. If desired, add more rosemary and drizzle with olive oil over the tops.

Bake for twenty to twenty-five minutes or until browned. Before serving, allow it to cool slightly.

Nutritional Information

Calories: 150

Carbohydrates: 22g

Protein: 3g

Fat: 5g

Fiber: 1g

Sodium: 120mg

Sun-Kissed Harvest

Yield: 1 large loaf, about 10 slices

Prep: 20 mins, Rise: 4-6 hours, baking: 45 mins)

Ingredients:

Flours: equal parts brown rice and millet flour (1 ½ cups each)

Dry: 1 tsp yeast, 1 ½ tsp salt

Wet: 1 tbsp honey, 1 ¼ cup warm water

Toppings: chopped sun-dried tomatoes, roasted zucchini, Kalamata olives (all ¼ cup)

Herbs: ½ tsp dried thyme

Instructions:

In a large basin, whisk together the dry trio of flour, salt, and yeast.

Beat the honey into the heated water in another basin. Stir the olives, thyme, and chopped veggies into the water mixture.

Stir until a dough forms by pouring the wet components into the dry ones. For four to six hours, or until doubled in size, cover and let rise at room temperature.

Set oven temperature to 200°C or 400°F. Put parchment paper on one baking sheet.

Roll the dough into a round loaf. Scorch the top with a sharp knife after transferring it to the baking sheet that has been prepared.

Bake for forty-five minutes, or until the top is golden brown and a toothpick inserted in the centre comes out clean. Before slicing, allow it to cool on a wire rack.

Nutritional Information:

Per slice (assuming 10 slices):

Calories: 240

Carbohydrates: 35g

Protein: 5g

Fat: 7g

Fiber: 3g

Sodium: 300mg

Honey Oat & Apple Spice

Yield: 1 large loaf, about 10 slices

Prep: 20 mins, Rise: 4-6 hours, baking: 45 mins)

Ingredients:

Flours: equal parts oat and buckwheat flour (1 cup each)

Dry: 1 tsp yeast, 1.5 tsp salt

Wet: 1 tbsp honey, 1.25 cup warm water

Apple: 1 grated apple

Spices: 1 tsp ground cinnamon, 0.25 tsp ground nutmeg

Directions:

Begin by whisking the flour, yeast, and salt together in a large bowl.

In another bowl, mix warm water and honey. Grated apple, nutmeg, and cinnamon should be added to the water mixture.

Mix until a dough forms, then pour the wet components into the dry ingredients. Once it has doubled in size, cover it and let it rise at room temperature for four to six hours.

Ensure that you preheat the oven to 400°F (200 °C) and prep your baking sheet with parchment paper.

Form the dough into a circular loaf very gently. Transfer to the prepared baking sheet and score the top with a sharp knife.

Bake for forty-five minutes, or until the top is golden brown and a toothpick inserted in the centre comes out clean. Before slicing, allow it to cool on a wire rack.

Nutritional Information:

Per slice (assuming 10 slices):

Calories: 220

Carbohydrates: 32g

Protein: 4g

Fat: 3g

Fiber: 4g

Sodium: 250mg

Smoked Cheddar & Scallion Surprise

Yield: 1 large loaf, about 10 slices

Prep: 15 mins, Rise: 4-6 hours, baking: 45 mins)

Ingredients:

Flours: A blend of 1 ½ cups spelt and ½ cup sorghum.

Leavening: 1 teaspoon active dry yeast.

Seasoning: 1 ½ teaspoons salt and 1 tablespoon honey.

Liquid: 1 ¼ cup warm water.

Toppings: ½ cup grated smoked cheddar cheese and ¼ cup chopped scallions.

Directions:

In a large basin, combine the dry base: flour, yeast, and salt.

In another bowl, mix warm water and honey. To the water mixture, add grated cheese and sliced scallions.

Mix until a dough is formed, and pour the wet components into the dry ingredients. On a surface dusted with flour, knead for five minutes.

Cover and let it rise at room temperature for 4-6 hours or until it is doubled in size.

Set a baking sheet with parchment paper and ensure to preheat the oven to 400°F (200°C).

Gently cradle the dough and fold it in on itself a few times to create a taut surface. Place it seam-side down on the baking sheet and score it with a classic X pattern.

Bake for 45 minutes or until golden brown with a clean toothpick test. Cool on a wire rack before slicing.

Nutrition information:

Per slice (assuming 10 slices):

Calories: 260

Carbohydrates: 34g

Protein: 7g

Fat: 8g

Fiber: 3g

Sodium: 350mg

Cranberry Orange Zest Celebration

Yield: 1 large loaf, about 10 slices

Prep: 20 mins, Rise: 4-6 hours, baking: 45 mins)

Ingredients:

Flours: A blend of 1 1/2 cups brown rice flour and 1/2 cup sorghum flour.

Leavening: 1 teaspoon active dry yeast.

Seasoning: 1 1/2 teaspoons salt and one tablespoon honey.

Liquid: 1 1/4 cup warm water (90-95°F).

Cranberry topping: 1 cup chopped fresh cranberries, 1 tbsp grated orange zest, and 1/4 teaspoon ground cinnamon.

Directions:

Start your dough by mixing flour, yeast, and salt in a large container.

In another bowl, mix warm water and honey. To the water mixture, add cinnamon, orange zest, and cranberries.

Mix until a dough forms, then pour the wet components into the dry ingredients. Once it has doubled in size, cover it and let it rise at room temperature for four to six hours.

Prep the oven: 400°F (200°C) and line a baking sheet.

To equally distribute the cranberries and orange zest, gently fold the dough. Form the dough into a circle and gently transfer it to the ready baking sheet.

Bake for 45 minutes or until golden brown with a clean toothpick test. Cool on a wire rack before slicing.

Nutritional Information:

Per slice (assuming 10 slices):

Calories: 230

Carbohydrates: 33g

Protein: 3g

Fat: 5g

Fiber: 4g

Sodium: 220mg

Roasted Veggie Rainbow

Yield: 1 large loaf, about 10 slices

Prep: 25 mins, Rise: 4-6 hours, baking: 45 mins)

Ingredients:

Flours: Equal parts almond and teff flour (1 cup each)

Leavening: 1 teaspoon yeast

Seasoning: 1 ½ teaspoons salt and 1 tablespoon honey

Liquid: 1 ¼ cup warm water

Roasted vegetables: ½ cup diced carrots, ½ cup diced bell peppers, and ¼ cup diced zucchini

Fresh herbs (optional): 1-2 tablespoons chopped basil or parsley

Directions:

Get your oven ready by preparing it to 400°F (200 °C). Don't forget to line a baking sheet with parchment paper for easy cleanup!

Toss dry ingredients: flour, yeast, and salt in a large bowl.

In another bowl, mix warm water and honey. To the water mixture, add the roasted veggies and fresh herbs, if using.

Mix until a dough forms, then pour the wet components into the dry ingredients. On a surface dusted with flour, knead for five minutes.

Once it has doubled in size, cover it and let it rise at room temperature for four to six hours.

Gently shape the dough into a circular loaf, nestle it on the baking sheet, and score the top with a knife.

Bake for 45 minutes or until golden brown. Check doneness with a toothpick in the centre; it should come out clean. Cool on a rack before slicing.

Nutritional Information:

Per slice (assuming 10 slices):

Calories: 210

Carbohydrates: 30g

Protein: 4g

Fat: 7g

Fiber: 3g

Sodium: 200mg

CHAPTER 4

Baguette Bliss: Mastering Crispy, Airy Baguettes

Classic Parisian Baguette

Yield: 2 baguettes, 8 slices each

Prep: 15 mins, Rise: 2-3 hours, Bake: 20-25 mins)

Ingredients:

Bread flour: 1 ½ cups

Tapioca & potato starch: ½ cup each

Yeast: 1 tsp

Salt: 1 ½ tsp

Cool water: ~1 ½ cups

Directions:

Carefully Mix flour, yeast, and salt in a large bowl. As you mix, gradually add water until a shaggy dough develops. On a lightly floured surface, knead for ten minutes or until the dough is smooth and elastic.

After putting the dough in a greased basin, cover it and leave it to rise for two to three hours or until it has doubled in size.

Prepare the oven to 450°F (230°C), and if using, prepare the baking stone as well. Split the dough into two halves, then form each into a long, thin baguette.

At a 45-degree angle, score the top of each baguette with sharp diagonal slashes. Spread out on a baking stone or sheet.

Bake for 20 to 25 minutes or until crusty and golden brown. Chill on a cooling rack prior to slicing.

Nutritional Information:

Per slice (assuming 8 slices per baguette):

Calories: 150

Carbohydrates: 28g

Protein: 3g

Fat: 1g

Fiber: 1g

Sodium: 200mg

Sesame & Poppy Seed Twists

Yield: 12 rolls

Prep: 15 mins, Rise: 2-3 hours, Bake: 20-25 mins)

Ingredients:

Same as Classic Parisian Baguette +

¼ cup each of sesame seeds and poppy seeds

Instructions:

Follow steps 1-3 from the Classic Parisian Baguette recipe.

Separate the dough into 12 equal halves. Each component should be rolled into a 12-inch-long rope.

Brush with water and sprinkle with a mixture of sesame and poppy seeds. Loosely wind each rope into a knot.

Knots should be transferred to a parchment paper-lined baking sheet.

Bake for twenty to twenty-five minutes or until browned.

Nutritional Information:

Per roll:

Calories: 120

Carbohydrates: 23g

Protein: 2g

Fat: 3g

Fiber: 1g

Sodium: 150mg

Garlic Parmesan Knots

Yield: 12 knots

Prep: 20 mins, Rise: 2-3 hours, Bake: 20-25 mins)

Ingredients:

Garlic butter: 2 tbsp melted butter mixed with 2 minced garlic cloves.

Parmesan boost: ½ cup grated Parmesan cheese.

Fresh touch (optional): Chopped parsley.

Directions:

As directed in the Classic Parisian Baguette recipe, follow steps 1-3.

Separate the dough into 12 equal halves. Each component should be rolled into a 12-inch-long rope.

Drizzle with melted butter, then top with Parmesan cheese and garlic. Make a knot out of each rope.

Knots should be transferred to a parchment paper-lined baking sheet. Bake for twenty to twenty-five minutes or until browned.

Before serving, garnish with chopped parsley (Optional)

Nutritional Information:

Per knot:

Calories: 180

Carbohydrates: 28g

Protein: 4g

Fat: 7g

Fiber: 1g

Sodium: 250mg

Herb-Infused Olive Twigs

Yield: 15-20 twigs

Prep: 20 mins, Rise: 2-3 hours, Bake: 20-25 mins

Ingredients:

Same as Classic Parisian Baguette +

2 tbsp olive oil

2 tbsp chopped fresh rosemary

2 tbsp chopped fresh thyme

1 tbsp chopped fresh oregano

Directions:

Follow steps 1-3 from the Classic Parisian Baguette recipe.

Cut dough into 15–20 equal pieces. Each piece should be rolled into a thin, 8-inch-long rope.

Garnish with a blend of oregano, thyme, and rosemary and drizzle with olive oil.

Each rope should be twisted into a spiral that resembles an olive branch.

Place the twigs on a parchment paper-lined baking sheet. Bake for twenty to twenty-five minutes or until browned.

Nutritional Information:

Per twig:

Calories: 100

Carbohydrates: 20g

Protein: 2g

Fat: 3g

Fiber: 1g

Sodium: 120mg

Cranberry Orange Swirl Baguette

Yield: 1 baguette, 8 slices

Prep: 20 mins, Rise: 2-3 hours, Bake: 20-25 mins

Ingredients:

Same as Classic Parisian Baguette +

½ cup chopped fresh cranberries

1 tbsp orange zest

¼ cup sugar

Directions:

Just follow the Classic Parisian Baguette recipe's first three stages.

Split the dough into two halves. Mix orange zest and cranberries into one-half of the dough.

Divide the dough in half and roll each half into a rectangle. Place the orange-cranberry dough on top of the plain dough and roll up tightly.

After transferring onto a parchment paper-lined baking sheet, score the top.

Be sure to bake for 20 to 25 minutes or until golden brown. Prior to slicing, allow it to cool slightly.

Nutritional Information:

Per slice:

Calories: 170

Carbohydrates: 30g

Protein: 3g

Fat: 1g

Fiber: 1g

Sodium: 200mg

Chapter 5

Sun-Kissed Mediterranean Focaccia

Yield: 1 medium focaccia, 8-10 servings

Prep: 20 mins, Rise: 2-3 hours, Bake: 30-35 mins

Ingredients:

Flours: 3 cups all-purpose

Leavening: 1 teaspoon active dry yeast

Seasoning: 1 ½ teaspoons salt, 1 tablespoon olive oil

Liquid: 1 ¼ cups warm water

Toppings: ½ cup chopped sun-dried tomatoes, ¼ cup chopped Kalamata olives, 1 tablespoon chopped fresh rosemary

Drizzle: Additional olive oil

Directions:

Carefully combine the flour, yeast, and salt in a large bowl. Mix in warm water and olive oil until a dough is formed. On a floured surface, knead the dough for ten minutes or until it is elastic and smooth.

Put the dough in a bowl that has been oiled, cover it, and let it rise for two to three hours or until it has doubled in size.

Prep the oven to 425°F (220°C) and slick a baking sheet with olive oil.

Spread out the dough into a thick rectangle by pressing it onto the baking sheet.

Using your fingertips, create dimples in the dough. Add sun-dried tomatoes, rosemary, and olives on top. Drizzle in a little more olive oil.

Bake for 30 to 35 minutes or until crusty and golden brown. Before slicing and serving, allow it to cool slightly.

Nutritional Information:

Per serving (assuming 8 slices):

Calories: 300

Carbohydrates: 45g

Protein: 6g

Fat: 10g

Fiber: 3g

Sodium: 350mg

Roasted Garlic & Fig Focaccia

Yield: 1 small focaccia, 6-8 servings

Prep: 25 mins, Rise: 2-3 hours, Bake: 30-35 mins)

Ingredients:

Garlic: 2 cloves, sliced thin

Oil: 1 tablespoon olive oil

Jam: 1/4 cup fig jam

Walnuts: 1/4 cup chopped (optional)

Directions:

Follow through steps 1-2 of the recipe for Sun-Kissed Mediterranean Focaccia.

Turn the oven on to 400°F or 200°C. Garlic slices should be tossed in olive oil and baked for 15 minutes or until they turn brown and caramelize.

Press the dough evenly onto a baking sheet. Over the dough, apply patches of fig jam. Add a layer of caramelized garlic over top and, if desired, sprinkle walnuts on top.

Bake for 30 to 35 minutes or until crusty and golden brown. Before slicing and serving, allow it to cool slightly.

Nutritional Information:

Per serving (assuming 8 slices):

Calories: 350

Carbohydrates: 48g

Protein: 5g

Fat: 13g

Fiber: 4g

Sodium: 320mg

Caramelized Onion & Smoked Gouda

Focaccia Yield: 1 medium focaccia, 8-10 servings

Prep: 30 mins, Rise: 2-3 hours, Bake: 30-35 mins

Ingredients:

Same as Sun-Kissed Mediterranean Focaccia +

2 large onions, thinly sliced

2 tbsp olive oil

1/4 cup water

1/4 cup crumbled smoked Gouda cheese

1 tsp fresh thyme leaves

Directions:

Follow steps 1-2 of the recipe for Sun-Kissed Mediterranean Focaccia.

Turn the oven on to 400°F or 200°C. Garlic slices should be tossed in olive oil and baked for 15 minutes or until they turn brown and caramelize.

Press the dough evenly onto a baking sheet. Over the dough, apply patches of fig jam. Add a layer of caramelized garlic over top and, if desired, scatter walnuts on top.

Bake for 30 to 35 minutes or until crusty and golden brown. Before slicing and serving, allow it to cool a bit.

Nutritional Information:

Per serving (assuming 8 slices):

Calories: 320

Carbohydrates: 47g

Protein: 7g

Fat: 12g

Fiber: 3g

Sodium: 400mg

Herb Garden Loaf

Yield: 1 large loaf, 10-12 slices

Prep: 10 mins, Rise: 12-16 hours, Bake: 45-50 mins

Ingredients:

Floury base: 3 cups bread flour, 1 cup lively sourdough starter

Savory blend: 1 1/2 tsp salt, 1/4 cup each of chopped fresh parsley, basil, oregano, and thyme

Instructions:

In a large basin, mix flour, salt, and sourdough starter. Stir to produce a shaggy dough. Add the herbs and knead until smooth, about 5 minutes, on a surface dusted with flour.

Transfer dough to an oiled basin, cover it, and let it rise for 12 to 16 hours at room temperature or until doubled.

Prep the oven to about 400°F, or 200°C. Transfer the dough ball, rounded side down, to a baking sheet. Score the top with a sharp knife.

Bake for 45 to 50 minutes or until golden brown and crusty. Let cool completely before slicing and arranging.

Nutritional Information:

Per slice (assuming 10 slices):

Calories: 200

Carbohydrates: 38g

Protein: 5g

Fat: 2g

Fiber: 3g

Sodium: 250mg

Spicy Jalapeno Popper Focaccia

Yield 12 squares

Prep: 20 mins, Rise: 2-3 hours, Bake: 25-30 mins)

Ingredients:

Spicy topping: 1 jalapeno pepper, thinly sliced

Creamy contrast: ¼ cup softened cream cheese

Melty goodness: ¼ cup shredded cheddar cheese

Freshness boost (optional): 1 tbsp chopped fresh cilantro

Directions:

Carefully combine the flour, yeast, and salt in a large bowl. Mix in warm water and olive oil until a dough is formed. On a floured surface, knead the dough for ten minutes or until it is elastic and smooth.

Put the dough in a bowl that has been oiled, cover it, and let it rise for two to three hours or until it has doubled in size.

Aim for 425°F (220°C) in the oven. If you want a softer taste, you may sauté the jalapeño slices in a skillet; if you want a greater kick, you can leave them raw.

Press the dough into squares by placing it on a baking pan. On each square, spread some cream cheese. Add slices of jalapeño and grated cheddar cheese on top.

Bake for 25 to 30 minutes, until the cheese is bubbling and melted and the crust is golden brown.

Be sure that before serving, allow it to cool slightly and top with freshly chopped cilantro (optional).

Nutritional Information:

Per square (assuming 12 squares):

Calories: 250

Carbohydrates: 38g

Protein: 6g

Fat: 10g

Fiber: 2g

Sodium: 300mg

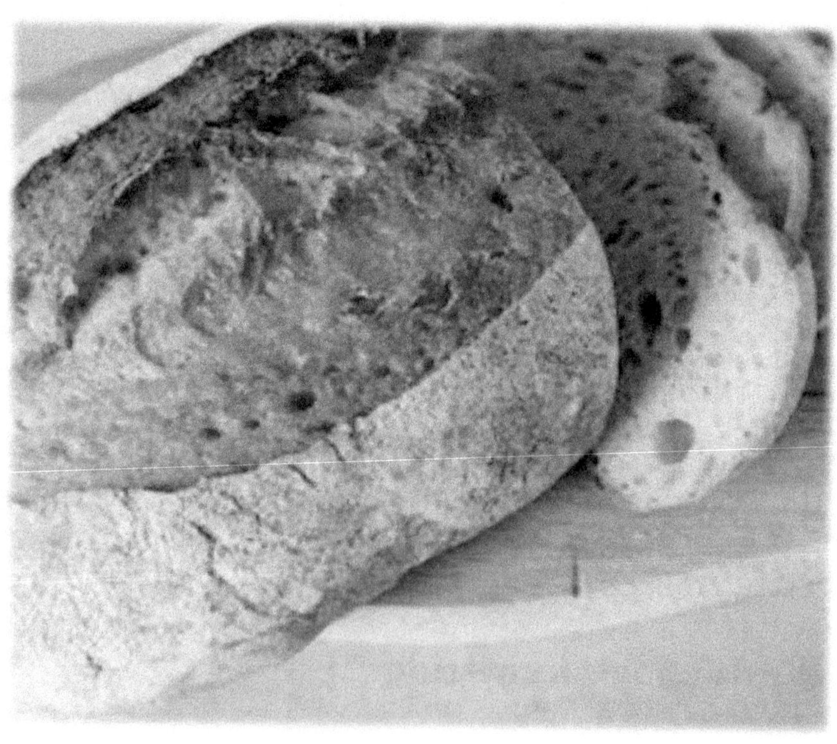

CHAPTER 6

Pizza Perfection and Beyond

Classic Neapolitan Dough

Yield: 2 pizzas, 4-6 servings each

Prep: 10 mins, Rest: 8-10 hours, Bake: 90 seconds

Ingredients:

Base: 500g fine-milled, low-protein Tipo 00 flour

Leavening: 8g active dry yeast

Hydration: 350ml lukewarm water

Flavor: 12g sea salt, 1 tbsp olive oil

Instructions:

Combine flour and yeast in a bowl. Add the dissolved salt to the flour mixture. Knead until elastic and smooth, approximately 10 minutes.

After putting the dough in a lightly oiled basin, cover it and let it rise at room temperature for eight to ten hours.

Preheat the oven to 450°C (840°F) and ensure to place a baking sheet or pizza stone on the lowest rack.

Split the dough into two halves, then carefully roll each into a thin circle on a surface dusted with flour.

Add a dab of olive oil, fior di latte mozzarella, and San Marzano tomatoes on top.

Preheat the pizza stone or baking sheet and bake for 90 seconds or until the crust is bubbly and brown.

Nutritional information (per pizza slice):

Calories: 250

Carbohydrates: 40g

Protein: 8g

Fat: 7g

Fiber: 2g

Sodium: 300mg

Biga-Fermented Neapolitan

Yield: 2-3 pizzas

Total Time: 20-24 hours)

Ingredients:

Biga:

Fine flour: 100 grams (Tipo 00 recommended)

Yeast: Pinch (about 0.5 grams active dry yeast)

Water: 60 millilitres (lukewarm)

Salt: 2 grams (sea salt preferred)

Main Dough:

Fine flour: 400 grams (Tipo 00 recommended)

Water: 280 millilitres (lukewarm)

Salt: 8 grams (sea salt preferred)

Olive oil: 1 tablespoon

Directions:

Biga: Put all of the ingredients for biga in a bowl. Cover and leave to rise for 12 to 16 hours at room temperature.

Main Dough: In a large basin, whisk together flour and yeast. Stir in the raised biga, salt, olive oil, and the remaining water. Until elastic and smooth, knead for ten minutes.

Rise and Shape: Cover the dough in an oiled basin and let it rise for two to three hours. Avoid overworking the dough as you gently stretch it into thin pizzas.

Top and Bake: Proceed with your favorite Neapolitan topping and baking directions, being sure to preheat the oven to a high temperature (450°C, 840°F) for a short bake time (90 seconds).

Nutritional Information (per slice, assuming 3 pizzas): Calories: 250, Carbohydrates: 35g

Protein: 6g

Fat: 7g

Fiber: 2g

Whole-Wheat Neapolitan

Yield: 2 pizzas

Total Time: 8-10 hours

Ingredients:

Flours: Equal parts Tipo 00 and whole-wheat flour (250g each).

Wet: 350ml lukewarm water, 1 tbsp olive oil.

Leavening: 8g active dry yeast.

Seasoning: 12g sea salt.

Directions:

Toss the flour and yeast together in a mixing bowl. Incorporate the dissolved salt into the flour mixture. Add olive oil and knead for ten minutes.

Rise and Shape: To rise, put the dough in an oiled basin, cover it, and let it be there for eight to ten hours. Stretch into thin pizzas very gently.

Top and Bake: Proceed with the topping of your choice and bake as directed, being sure to use a high oven temperature (450°C, 840°F) for a quick baking time (90 seconds).

Nutritional Information (per slice, assuming 2 pizzas): Calories: 230

Carbohydrates: 33g

Protein: 6g

Fat: 6g

Fiber: 2.5g

Gluten-Free Neapolitan

Yield; 1-2 pizzas

Total Time: 2.5 hours)

Ingredients:

Gluten-free flours: A trifecta of almond, tapioca, and brown rice flours (150g each).

Leavening: 8g active dry yeast, activated in 300ml lukewarm water.

Dry ingredients: 2g xanthan gum, 1/4 tsp baking soda, and 1/4 tsp salt.

Fat: 1 tbsp olive oil.

Directions:

In a bowl, combine the dry ingredients. Mix the water-dissolved yeast with the dry ingredients. Work dough for five minutes while adding olive oil.

Rise and Shape: Put the dough into a covered, oiled basin and allow it to rise for two hours. Stretch into thin pizzas very gently.

Top and Bake: Bake for 10 to 12 minutes, ensuring the bottom crust is crisp at 400°C (750°F).

Nutritional information (per slice, assuming 2 pizzas): Calories: 210

Carbohydrates: 30g

Protein: 4g

Fat: 7g

Fiber: 2g

Rosemary and Sea Salt Neapolitan

Yield: 2-3 pizzas

Total Time: 8-10 hours)

Ingredients:

Flour: 500g Tipo 00 (the foundation)

Leavening: 8g active dry yeast (for a beautiful rise)

Liquid: 350ml lukewarm water (to bring it all together)

Seasoning: 12g sea salt (for savory depth)

Olive oil: 1 tbsp (for richness and texture)

Fresh aromatics: 1 sprig of fresh rosemary, chopped (a touch of herbal elegance, optional)

Directions:

Classic Dough: Combine flour and yeast in a large bowl. Add the dissolved salt to the flour mixture. Knead until elastic and smooth, approximately 10 minutes.

Rosemary Infusion (Optional): Finely slice a rosemary sprig for a light herbal scent and mix it into the dough while it is being kneaded.

Rise and Shape: put the dough in an oiled basin, cover it, and let it rise for eight to ten hours. Stretch the dough gently into thin pizzas, careful not to overwork it.

Salted Finish (Optional): To provide a great texture and flavor contrast, sprinkle crushed sea salt over the stretched dough.

Top and Bake: Proceed with the topping of your choice and bake as directed, being sure to use a high oven temperature (450°C, 840°F) for a quick baking time (90 seconds).

Nutritional Information (per slice, assuming 2 pizzas):

Calories: 250

Carbohydrates: 35g

Protein: 6g

Fat: 7g

Fiber: 2g

Beyond the Round

Get rid of the sphere's predicted perfection and the circle's tyranny! Shapes in the doughy world of bread are more than simply visual appeal; they open doors to gastronomic possibilities, with every fold, twist, and incision holding a narrative just waiting to be told. Now, take out your rolling pin, let your inner sculptor loose, and get ready to go on an adventure into the realm of bread that goes beyond the round loaf.

Braided Beauties:

Braids are the ballerinas of the bread world. They appear in everything from the golden challah with its arms entwined in a symbol of oneness to the flaky Danish pastry with its buttery whisper of luxury in its lattice layers. Because of their layered structure, which creates pockets for fillings, they become enticing visual displays that may be decorated with an infinite variety of savory or sweet surprises.

Folded Delights:

Picture a book with pockets of melted cheese and layers of buttery bread instead of text. Like a light French croissant, the folded bread's exquisite layers are a monument to the baker's skill. That's what makes it magical. Alternatively, consider the modest Stromboli, the Italian cousin of the calzone, with its crescent-shaped crust and savory ingredients ideal for on-the-go munching.

Knots of Flavor:

Intricate forms made of dough that are enjoyable to produce and devour are known as knots, the mischievous pranksters of the bread world. A typical example is the pretzel, which has a chewy inside and a salty outside but does take into account the adaptability of the knot.

Many more kinds are still waiting to be discovered, including cheesy knots bursting with mozzarella or garlic knots sprinkled with delicious herb butter.

Flatbread Fiesta:

From the sun-drenched shores of the Mediterranean comes the focaccia, a canvas of golden dough begging to be adorned with olives, tomatoes, and herbs. In India, the soft and pillowy naan gracefully cradles stews and sauces. Furthermore, in Mexico, the tortilla—a blank canvas of delicious cornmeal—becomes the medium for tacos, quesadillas, and many other culinary creations.

Bread Sculptures:

Bread is an art form as well as a food source. Expert bakers can create amazing sculptures out of dough, ranging from elaborate flowers and animals to fantastical castles and life-size portraits. These delectable works of art demonstrate the infinite inventiveness of the human spirit and demonstrate that bread can serve as both nourishment and art and as a catalyst for debate.

So embrace the countless variations in bread forms and break free from the monotony of round loaves. Explore your creative side, try out folds, twists, and braids, and go beyond the conventional circle to uncover a flavorful and enjoyable world. Remember that bread is more than simply food; it's an artistic medium, a vehicle for conversation, and a gastronomic adventure meant to be enjoyed one mouthful at a time.

CHAPTER 7

Sweet Treats with Sourdough

Tangy Dream Cinnamon Rolls

Yield: 12

Total Time: 4 hours:

Ingredients:

Dough:

1 cup bubbly sourdough starter (227g)

3/4 cup creamy milk (170g)

1 large egg

4 tablespoons softened butter (57g)

Flours: 2 3/4 cups all-purpose (330g) + 1/2 cup whole wheat (57g)

Sweetness & salt: 1/4 cup granulated sugar (50g) + 1 1/2 teaspoons salt

Filling:

Spiced crumble: 3/4 cup light brown sugar (159g) + 1/4 cup flour (30g) + 1 tablespoon cinnamon + 1/8 teaspoon salt, mixed with 1 tablespoon melted butter

Glaze:

Sweet & creamy: 1 1/2 cups powdered sugar (170g) + pinch salt, whipped with 1 1/2 tablespoons softened butter and 1/2 teaspoon vanilla extract, thinned with 1-2 tablespoons milk.

Directions:

Make dough: combine starter, milk, egg, butter, flour, sugars, and salt. Knead for 10 minutes. Rise for 2 hours.

Combine brown sugar, flour, cinnamon, and salt to fill. Roll out the dough, top with filling, slice, and roll up. Toss in a pan and let rise for an hour.

Be sure to bake for approximately 20 to 25 minutes at 375°F (190°C). Glaze recipe in ingredients.

Nutritional Information (per roll):

Calories: 350

Carbohydrates: 45g

Protein: 5g

Fat: 15g

Fiber: 3g.

Citrus Burst Lemon Cookies

Yield: 24

Total Time: 1 hour:

Ingredients:

Lively starter and creamy base:

1 cup (227g) active sourdough starter

1/2 cup (113g) softened butter

Sweetness and citrus zest:

3/4 cup (150g) sugar

1 large egg

1 teaspoon lemon zest

1/4 cup (60ml) lemon juice

Classic foundation:

2 1/2 cups (310g) all-purpose flour

1 teaspoon baking powder

1/2 teaspoon salt

Directions:

Cream butter and sugar, beat in egg, zest, and juice. Stir in baking powder, salt, flour, and starter. Let the dough cool for half an hour.

Turn the oven on to 375°F, or 190°C. Place dough on baking pans and bake for ten to twelve minutes.

Nutritional Information (per cookie):

Calories: 150

Carbohydrates: 20g

Protein: 1g

Fat: 7g

Fiber: 1g.

Sourdough Stack Pancakes

Yield: 6

Total Time: 30 minutes):

Ingredients:

One cup (227g) active sourdough starter & 1 cup (240ml) buttermilk (tangy base)

1 egg, 1 tbsp honey & 1 tbsp melted butter (wet & sweet)

One and a half cups (187g) of all-purpose flour, one and a half teaspoons of baking powder, and half a teaspoon of flaky, dry salt.

Directions:

Whisk starter, buttermilk, egg, honey, and butter. In another bowl, combine the dry ingredients. Combine the dry and wet ingredients, whisking just until blended.

Be sure to heat your pan or griddle to a medium temperature. Cook pancakes until both sides are golden brown.

Nutritional Information (per pancake):

Calories: 200

Carbohydrates: 25g

Protein: 5g

Fat: 7g

Fiber: 2g.

Cozy Sourdough Coffee Cake

Yield: 8-10

Total time: 2 hours

Ingredients:

Cake:

Flours: 2.5 cups combined (2 all-purpose, 0.5 whole-wheat)

Leaveners: 1.5 tsp baking powder, 0.5 tsp baking soda

Wet: Half (1/2) cup softened butter, One (1) cup sugar, two eggs, 1 cup milk, 0.5 cup sour cream, 0.5 cup sourdough starter

Seasoning: 0.5 tsp salt

Crumble:

Dry: 0.5 cup flour, 0.25 cup rolled oats, 0.25 cup brown sugar, 0.25 tsp cinnamon

Wet: 0.25 cup softened butter

Directions:

Prep: Preheat your oven to approximately 350°F (175°C) and grease/flour a 9x13 pan.

Dry: Mix cake flours, leaveners, and salt in a bowl.

Wet: Cream butter & sugar, then beat in eggs.

Combine: Alternate dry & wet ingredients with milk/sour cream/starter. Mix just until combined. Pour batter into pan.

Crumble: Combine crumble ingredients and sprinkle over batter.

Bake: Be sure to bake for 50-60 minutes or until the toothpick comes out clean.

Nutritional Information (per slice):

Calories: 350

Carbohydrates: 45g

Protein: 5g

Fat: 15g

Fiber: 3g

Sourdough Apple Pie with a Kick

Yield: 8-10

Total time: 2.5 hours

Ingredients:

Crust:

Floury base: 2 cups all-purpose flour & ½ tsp salt

Chilly fat: ½ cup cold unsalted butter

Icy binding: ¼ cup ice water

Tangy boost: 2 tbsp sourdough starter

Filling:

Apple stars (6-7): Granny Smith or Honey crisp recommended (tart & sweet)

Sugary duo: ¼ cup each brown & granulated sugar (richness & depth)

Thickening touch: 1 tbsp cornstarch (prevents mushiness)

Warm spices: ½ tsp cinnamon & ¼ tsp nutmeg (cozy aroma)

Citrusy lift: 1 tbsp lemon juice (balances sweetness)

Directions:

Make the crust: Pulse the flour and salt in a food processor. Add the cold butter and pulse until small crumbs form. Add ice water and starter, pulsing just until the dough comes together. Shape into a disk, cover with plastic wrap, and chill for half an hour.

Get the filler ready: Once apples are peeled and cored, slice them thinly. Mix in the spices, cornstarch, lemon juice, and sugars.

Turn the oven on to 400°F or 200°C. Roll out the dough on a floured surface and transfer it to a

9-inch pie pan. Pour in filling and dab with butter.

Cover the pie with another rolled-out dough or cut out decorative shapes. Trim edges, then dab with milk. Bake for 50–60 minutes or until the filling bubbles and the crust golden brown.

Nutritional Information (per slice):

Calories: 300

Carbohydrates: 40g

Protein: 3g

Fat: 12g

Fiber: 3g

Sourdough Glazed Doughnuts

Yield: 12

Total Time: 2.5 hours:

Ingredients:

Dough:

Flours: 3.5 cups combined (2 bread flour, 1.5 all-purpose)

Sweetener: 1/4 cup sugar

Seasoning: 1 tsp salt, 1/4 tsp active dry yeast

Liquids: 1/2 cup warmed milk, 1/4 cup sourdough starter, 1/4 cup vegetable oil

Frying: Extra vegetable oil (optional)

Glazing: Sugar (optional)

Directions:

In a bowl, combine the dry ingredients. Add yeast, starter, and milk. Ensure to Knead until smooth and elastic, about 10 minutes. Allow to rise for one to two hours.

Roll out dough on a floured surface to 1/2-inch thickness. Using a doughnut cutter, cut into doughnuts. Give it another 30 minutes to rise.

Heat oil to 350°F (175°C). Fry doughnuts and flip them once until golden. Drain on paper towels.

Use a milk mixture and powdered sugar glaze (optional).

Nutritional Information (per doughnut, without glaze):

Calories: 150

Carbohydrates: 20g

Protein: 3g

Fat: 6g

Fiber: 1g

Sourdough Snicker doodles

Yield: 12

Total Time: 1 hour

Ingredients:

Creamy Base:

1 (One) cup each softened butter & sugar

1 (One) egg & 1 tsp vanilla extract

Dry Mix:

2 (two) cups all-purpose flour

1/2 (half) tsp baking soda & 1/4 tsp salt

Tangy Twist:

1/4 cup sourdough starter

Cinnamon Topping:

1/3 cup cinnamon sugar

Directions:

Cream together the sugar and butter until it's soft and Pillowy. Add vanilla and egg, and beat.

Mix the sourdough starter with the dry ingredients. Stir until well blended after adding to the wet ingredients.

Craft the dough into playful spheres, then adorn them with a dusting of cinnamon sugar. Ensure to bake on a baking sheet until golden and fragrant, 10-12 minutes at 375°F

.**Nutritional Information** (per cookie):

Calories: 180

Carbohydrates: 25g

Protein: 2g

Fat: 9g

Fiber: 1g

Sourdough Brioche French toast

Yield: 2

Total Time: 45 minutes

Ingredients:

French toast:

Bread: 2 thick slices of sourdough brioche

Egg Mixture: 2 eggs, 1/2 cup milk, 1/4 (quarter) tsp vanilla extract, 1/4 (quarter) tsp cinnamon, pinch of salt

Frying: Butter

Toppings: Fresh fruit, syrup, or powdered sugar (optional)

Directions:

Whisk your eggs, milk, vanilla extract, cinnamon, and salt in a bowl.

Soak bread slices in mixture for 5 minutes.

Ensure the butter is heated in a skillet over medium heat. Fry soaked the bread until golden brown on both sides.

Serve with fresh fruit, syrup, or powdered sugar.

Nutritional Information (per serving):

Calories: 450

Carbohydrates: 50g

Protein: 20g

Fat: 25g

Fiber: 3g

Sourdough Monkey Bread with Pecans

Yield: 1 generous loaf, enough for 8-10 hungry souls

Total Time: 45 minutes

Ingredients

Dough:

1 (One) sourdough bread dough (homemade or store-bought)

Topping:

1/2 cup light brown sugar, packed

1/4 cup melted, browned butter

1/2 tsp ground cinnamon

1/4 tsp kosher salt

1/2 cup chopped pecans (optional, toasted)

Drizzle (optional):

Caramel sauce (homemade or store-bought)

Instructions:

Tear the sourdough dough into walnut-sized pieces, about bite-sized portions. Envision yourself as an imaginative baker, letting your inner beast loose on a tender, cloud-like dough. Welcome to your freedom!

Mix the cinnamon, salt, melted butter, and brown sugar in a large basin. This flavorful mix will be the playground for your dough nuggets.

Coat the shredded dough pieces equally by tossing them in the spiced sugar mixture. Now, carefully fold in the toasted nuts, if using, making sure they get to interact with all of the tasty bowl companions.

Grease a loaf pan and gently nestle the dough mixture inside. Place the pan in a warm area and let it rise for thirty minutes. Consider it your doughy buddies' warm sleepover, enabling them to gain even more plumpness and fluff.

Prep the oven temperature to 350°F (175°C). The dough should be baked for 30 to 35 minutes until the top is golden brown and the aroma of sweet, pure temptation wafts from it.

Drizzle some delicious caramel sauce over the warm monkey bread for an added layer of sticky-sweet perfection. Imagine the golden dough sparkling with jewel-like caramel; the sight and flavor are exquisite!

After letting the monkey bread cool for a few minutes, invite your loved ones for a pull-apart feast. A symphony of airy sourdough, crunchy nuts, and sweet caramel flavors will be present in every mouthful. Though you might be tempted to keep this lovely treasure to yourself, remember that sharing is caring!

Nutritional Information (per serving, without caramel sauce):

Calories: ~350

Carbohydrates: ~45g

Protein: ~5g

Fat: ~15g

Fiber: ~2g

Sourdough Croissants with Raspberry Filling

Yield: 10

Total Time: 4 hours

Ingredients:

Base:

1 (One) recipe of sourdough bread dough (homemade or store-bought)

Filling:

1/4 cup softened butter

1/4 cup sugar

1/4 teaspoon cinnamon

1/2 cup fresh raspberries

Topping:

Egg wash (1 (One) egg beaten with 1 (One) tablespoon water)

Directions:

Roll the sourdough dough out into a rectangle while it's cold. Apply butter that has softened.

Sprinkle with sugar and cinnamon. The dough is folded into thirds and rolled like a log.

Slice thickly and form into crescents. Transfer to a baking sheet, cover, and allow it to rise for one to two hours.

Brush with egg wash after stuffing raspberries into each croissant. Then, bake for about 15 to 20 minutes at 375°F (190°C) or until golden brown.

Nutritional Information (per croissant, without filling): Calories: 200

Carbohydrates: 25g

Protein: 3g

Fat: 9g

Fiber: 1g

Sourdough Banana Bread with Walnuts

Yield: 1 loaf

Total Time: 1.5 hours

Ingredients:

Sweet Trio: 3 mashed bananas, 1/4 cup each of oil & milk, 1 (One) egg, and 1 cup sourdough discard.

Flour Power: 1.5 cups combined flour (1 all-purpose, 0.5 whole wheat)

Rise & Shine: 0.5 tsp each baking soda & powder, 0.25 tsp salt

Nutty Crunch: 0.5 cup chopped walnuts

Directions:

Prep oven temperature to 175°C/350°F. Grease a loaf pan.

Mash bananas, oil, milk, egg, and sourdough discard should all be combined in a bowl.

Whisk the dry ingredients in another basin. Mix until barely mixed after adding to the wet ingredients.

Fold in walnuts. After filling the pan, pour batter into it and bake for 50–60 minutes, or until the toothpick inserted into the center comes clean.

Nutritional Information (per slice):

Calories: 200

Carbohydrates: 30g

Protein: 4g

Fat: 8g

Fiber: 3g

Sourdough Blueberry Muffins

Yield: 12

Total Time: 45 minutes

Ingredients:

Base: 1 cup each sourdough discard, milk, and all-purpose flour (equal parts)

Leavening & Seasoning: 2 tsp baking powder, 1/2 tsp salt

Wet: 1 egg, 1/4 cup each vegetable oil and sugar

Sweet Addition: 1 cup fresh blueberries

Directions:

Turn the oven on to 400°F or 200°C. Oil a muffin pan.

Whisk together oil, egg, milk, and sourdough discard in a bowl.

Fold dry ingredients into wet batter until just combined. Add the blueberries and fold.

Distribute batter among muffin cups. Bake for 15-20 minutes or until golden.

Nutritional Information (per muffin):

Calories: 200

Carbohydrates: 30g

Protein: 4g

Fat: 8g

Fiber: 2g

Sourdough Peach Cobbler with Ginger

Yield: 8-10 servings

Total Time: 1 hour

Ingredients:

Fruit Filling:

8 (Eight) juicy peaches, sliced

1/3 cup golden brown sugar

3 tbsp creamy butter

Spiced Dough:

2 cups all-purpose flour

1/4 cup sweet sugar

1 tsp baking powder

½ tsp salt

¼ cup tangy sourdough starter

½ cup creamy milk

Topping:

2 tbsp all-purpose flour

2 tsp warm cinnamon

⅛ tsp earthy nutmeg

½ tsp grated fresh ginger (or ¼ tsp ground)

⅓ Cup melted and cooled butter

Directions:

Turn the oven on to 400°F or 200°C. Combine brown sugar, butter, flour, nutmeg, nutcress, and ginger with peaches.

Mix dry topping ingredients in a bowl. Stir in milk, melted butter, and sourdough starter. Do not over mix; simply blend the ingredients.

Transfer the peach blend to a baking dish. Large dollops of cobbler dough should be dropped on top, leaving room in between.

Be sure to bake for 40 to 45 minutes, until bubbling and golden brown on top. Warm up and serve with whipped cream or ice cream (optional).

Nutritional Information (per serving, without ice cream):

Calories: ~350

Carbohydrates: ~50g

Protein: ~5g

Fat: ~15g

Fiber: ~2g

Sourdough Chocolate Babka

Yield: 1 loaf

Total Time: 4 hours

Ingredients:

Dough:

2 (Two) cups of bread flour

1/4 cup sugar

1 tsp salt

1/4 tsp active dry yeast

1/2 cup warmed milk

1/4 cup sourdough starter

1/4 cup softened butter

Filling & Finishing

1 egg

1 tsp vanilla extract

1 cup chocolate hazelnut spread

1 (One) egg yolk beaten with 1 tbsp milk (egg wash)

Flaked almonds or pearl sugar (optional)

Directions:

In a bowl, combine the dry ingredients to make the dough. Stir in yeast, starter, and milk. Knead for approximately ten minutes or until the dough is elastic and smooth. Allow to rise for one to two hours.

Make filling: Beat sugar, vanilla extract, and butter until frothy and light. Add chocolate-hazelnut spread and stir.

Assemble: Roll out dough into a rectangle. Evenly distribute filling over the top. Twist dough firmly from the long side, sealing ends with pinches. Twirl dough with three strands.

Place braided dough in a loaf pan, tucking ends under. Give it an hour to rise. Apply an egg wash coat and then scatter the topping (if desired).

Ensure to bake for approximately 45 to 50 minutes until golden brown at 350°F/175°C.

Before slicing and serving, allow it to cool slightly.

Nutritional Information (per slice):

Calories: ~400

Carbohydrates: ~50g

Protein: ~5g

Fat: ~20g

Fiber: ~2g

Sourdough Tiramisu Parfaits

Yield: 4-6 parfaits

Total Time: 1 hour

Ingredients:

Mascarpone Cream:

Creamy base: 1 cup mascarpone cheese

Sweetness: 1/4 cup powdered sugar

Tangy touch: 1/4 cup plain yogurt

Vanilla flair: 1/2 tsp vanilla extract

Pinch of salt

Coffee Soaking:

Espresso boost: 1 cup cooled strong coffee

Rum kick (optional): 2 tbsp rum

Chocolate depth: 1 tbsp cocoa powder

Ladyfingers:

Spongey base: 12-16 ladyfingers, broken

Toppings (optional):

Cocoa dusting

Chocolate shavings

Fresh berries

Directions:

Whip the Mascarpone Dream: In a mixing bowl, combine mascarpone cheese, powdered sugar, yogurt, vanilla extract, and salt. Whip until smooth and creamy. Set aside.

Coffee Infused Cocoa: Mix cooled coffee, rum (if using), and cocoa powder in a shallow dish. Dip ladyfinger pieces in the mixture to lightly coat, ensuring they don't become soggy.

Layered Delight: In individual glasses or parfait bowls, create layers of mascarpone cream, coffee-soaked ladyfingers, and a sprinkle of cocoa powder. Repeat until glasses are filled, ending with a final layer of mascarpone cream.

Chill and Charm: To let the flavors combine, and the ladyfingers soften even more, place the parfaits in the refrigerator for at least two hours.

Grand Finale: Before serving, dust with additional cocoa powder, grated chocolate, or fresh berries for an extra touch of elegance and flavor.

Nutritional Information (per parfait, without additional toppings):

Calories: ~300

Carbohydrates: ~35g

Protein: ~8g

Fat: ~15g

Fiber: ~2g

CHAPTER 8

The Art of Fermentation

Welcome, fellow bread enthusiasts, to the heart of the bakery, where dough dances with time and temperature, transforming humble ingredients into golden masterpieces. This chapter serves as your entryway into the intriguing world of shaping and fermentation, where the precise balance of heat, hands, and bacteria produces the ideal rise. Preheat your ovens, grab a seat, and let's go on an adventure that will take your bread-making to a whole new level.

Bulk Fermentation

Imagine your dough as a party of tiny yeast munching on sugar. They produce carbon dioxide bubbles, which cause the dough to inflate like a balloon. Meanwhile, some bacteria are busy creating delicious smells, whispering tang and depth. Not only does this enchanted gathering cause your bread to rise, but it also influences its taste and texture.

The temperature is like the music at this party. It sets the pace of the yeast dance: colder temperatures cause it to move more slowly. For the finest yeast party and a well-balanced flavor, aim for a comfortable temperature of 70–80°F (think summer breeze). Don't simply glance at the time, though! When your dough feels light and fluffy like a cloud and has doubled in size, it's ready to shape. The bread might become dense and gooey if the celebration lasts too long, much like a party that has lost its charm. So watch your dough and come to the party when the time is perfect!

Shaping: Sculpting the Dream Loaf

Okay, dough master! Now that your bread baby has grown like a pro, it's time to make it the center of attention. Shape without fear; see it as a conversation you can have with your dough, slowly forming it into the shape you choose. Just a little stretch and fold, twist and turn, like a tiny dance in the bakery, no roughhousing.

You'll be an expert at shaping bread after you get the hang of simple techniques like stretching it out, folding it over, or swirling it in a spiral pattern. The options are endless: you may create long, crispy baguettes, spherical loaves that resemble fluffy clouds, or anything in between! Let's begin shaping and exploring the wonder we can create with bread!

Bannet Bonanza: A Nest for Perfection

Instead of a boring bowl, give your dough a comfy "bannet" to snuggle up in while it rises. This comfortable nest keeps everything warm and content, allowing it to expand to its maximum capacity. A smooth, springy loaf that flaunts its beautiful shape in the oven is what you can expect.

Try experimenting with different flours and fancy "fluting" (a unique method of pinching the dough) to get a unique-looking loaf of bread. It's similar to creating a masterpiece out of simple dough! So, let your creative side come out and see how your invention rises to the occasion.

Baking Secrets for Golden Glories:

Imagine your oven as a fiery artist's studio, where dough gets sculpted into golden masterpieces. Let's play two key symphonies to unlock its secrets: Steam Symphony and Scoring Symphony.

Steam Symphony: Think of this as a spa day for your dough! A quick burst of steam early on creates a cozy, moist environment. Like a sun-kissed masterpiece, this helps your crust develop a gorgeous golden glow and shine. Just toss some ice cubes on your preheated baking stone, or give the oven walls a quick spritz with water – an instant steam bath!

Scoring Symphony: Those tiny slashes you see on bread? They're not just for show! They're like little breathing holes, helping your dough rise evenly and preventing it from cracking under pressure. So grab your favourite knife and get creative! Make swirls, lines, or even a checkerboard pattern – watch your dough blossom into a work of art as it bakes!

Troubleshooting: From Gummy to Glorious:

Even the most seasoned baker encounters challenges. But worry not—we have tools for troubleshooting!

Gummy Crumb: Over fermentation or under baking are common causes of this problem. Ensure your oven reaches the right temperature, check your rise, and modify the proofing timings.

Dense Texture: Dense loaves can be produced by overworking the dough or using excessive flour. Don't be afraid to experiment with hydration levels, modify flour ratios, and use mild shaping techniques.

Burnt Loaves: Ouch! This occurs when you bake for an excessive amount of time or when your oven is excessively hot. Reduce the oven's temperature a little, modify the baking duration according to the size of your loaf, and think about utilizing a baking stone to ensure even heating.

Baking is an adventure rather than a final goal. Accept that learning is a process, try out various methods, and don't be scared to get your hands dirty. Each flawed loaf serves as a springboard for the subsequent magnificent work of art. So, continue to study, explore, and bake your way to the pinnacle of bread excellence!

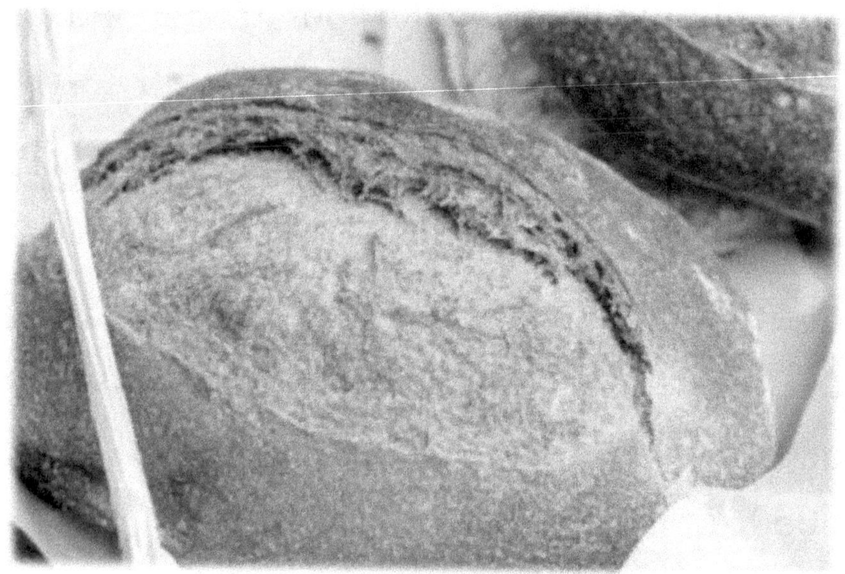

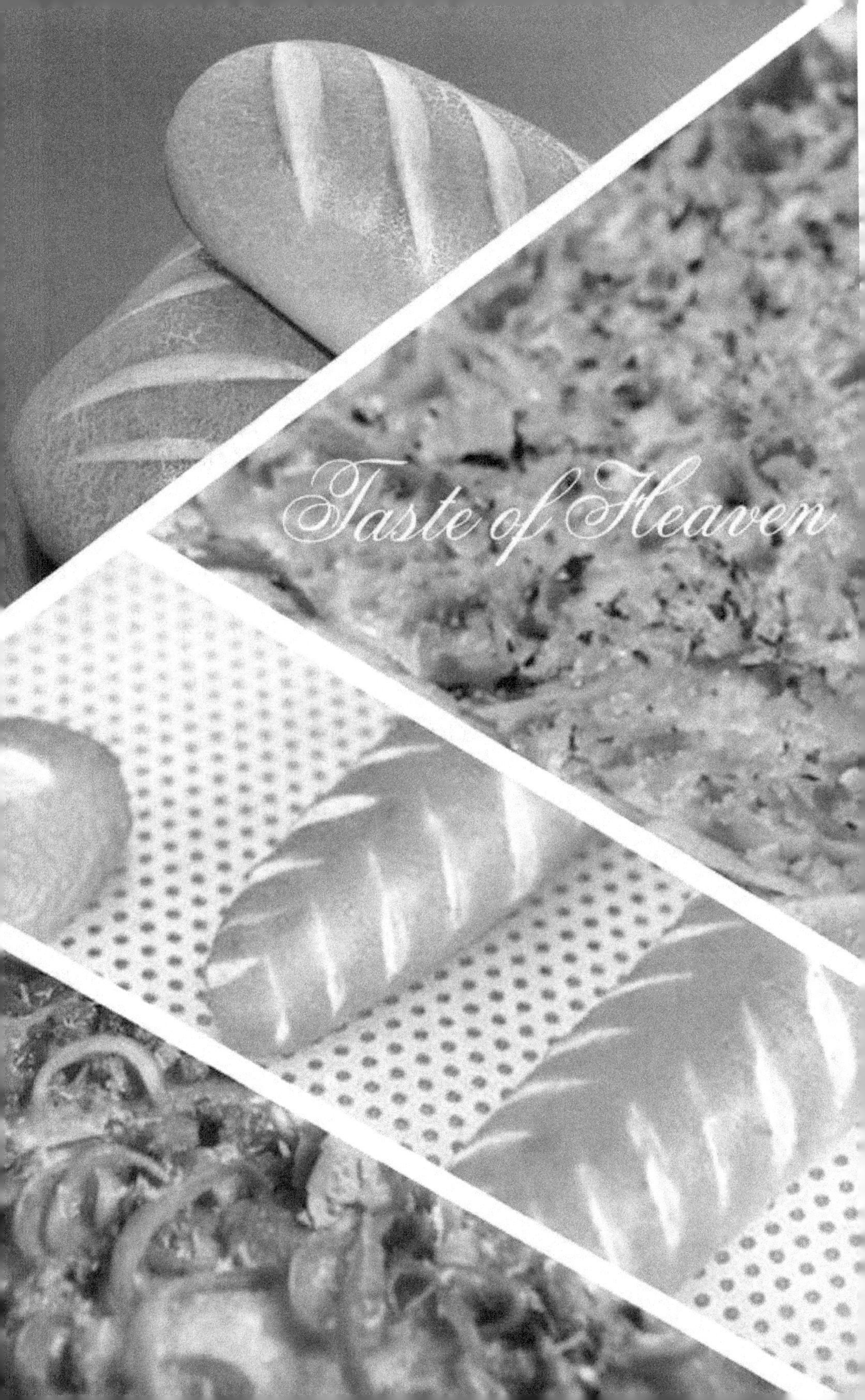
Taste of Heaven

CHAPTER 9

Sourdough Discard Magic

Do not be alarmed, fellow sourdough lovers! We've all had the familiar feeling when your bubbling starter flourishes and fills the jar to the brim, leaving you torn between discarding it and giving up. No more despair! We'll reveal the tricks of turning those leftover scraps into a delectable paradise of pancakes, waffles, crackers, and more in this chapter, your dedication to Sourdough Discard Magic!

Consider discards as fermented gold dust instead of trash. It's airy secrets, and tangy whispers have the power to give baked goods a depth and complexity never before seen. Fasten your seatbelts, preheat your ovens, and get ready to see your sourdough discard transform from ordinary leftovers into the focal point of your kitchen.

Pancakes of Pillowy Delight:

Imagine fluffy, golden pancakes infused with the subtle tang of sourdough. Discard gives them a magical touch that makes them lighter, more airy, and full of personality. To neutralize the acidity, include a small amount of sugar in your pancake mixture along with a small amount of baking soda. The result? Pancakes that soar like clouds and fill your palate with zesty delight.

Waffles Woven with Tang:

Elevate your waffle game with the power of discard! With each mouthful, the subtle acidity of it balances the sweetness of your batter, producing a symphony of flavors. Combine your leftovers with your regular waffle batter, allow it to sit for some extra fermentation, and then be ready to be blown away. You'll be yearning for more and more waffles as they come out of the iron, crisp and golden and full of flavor.

Crackers that Crunch with Character:

Craving a satisfyingly crunchy snack? Sourdough leftovers save the day! Crackers go well with its natural sharpness. Mix the discard into your cracker dough, add enough water to get the right texture, and see the magic happen. Bake them until golden and crisp, and experience the magic of discard crackling in your mouth with every satisfying bite.

Beyond the Breakfast Breadbasket:

Discard has much more magic than just breakfast foods. Give savory bread a deeper flavor by adding discard to focaccias, pizza dough's, and even rustic baguettes. Its subtle tang will go well with cheeses and savory additions to make very exceptional loaves.

Unleash your Inner Alchemist:

Always keep in mind that your journey with sourdough discard is just getting started! Try using discard in cakes, cookies, muffins, and flatbreads. See how its unique qualities work with various flours and sugars. You may be the one to create the next big breakfast trend!

A Few Words of Wisdom:

Discard Age: For pancakes and waffles, the younger Discard (3-5 days old) works best; for bread and crackers, the older Discard (7-10 days old) provides more tang.

Hydration: The degree of hydration in Discard can vary. If necessary, adjust your liquid proportions to get the proper dough consistency.

The acidity of sourdough requires balance. To get a well-balanced taste profile, add baking soda to pancakes and waffle batters and modify the amount of salt in other recipes.

So let go of your hopelessness and enjoy the magic! Your sourdough starter opens the door to a world of culinary adventures and is more than simply a bread maker. Proceed, try new things, and let your discard do its tart magic. Remember that a little leftover magic is what inspires inventiveness in the kitchen!

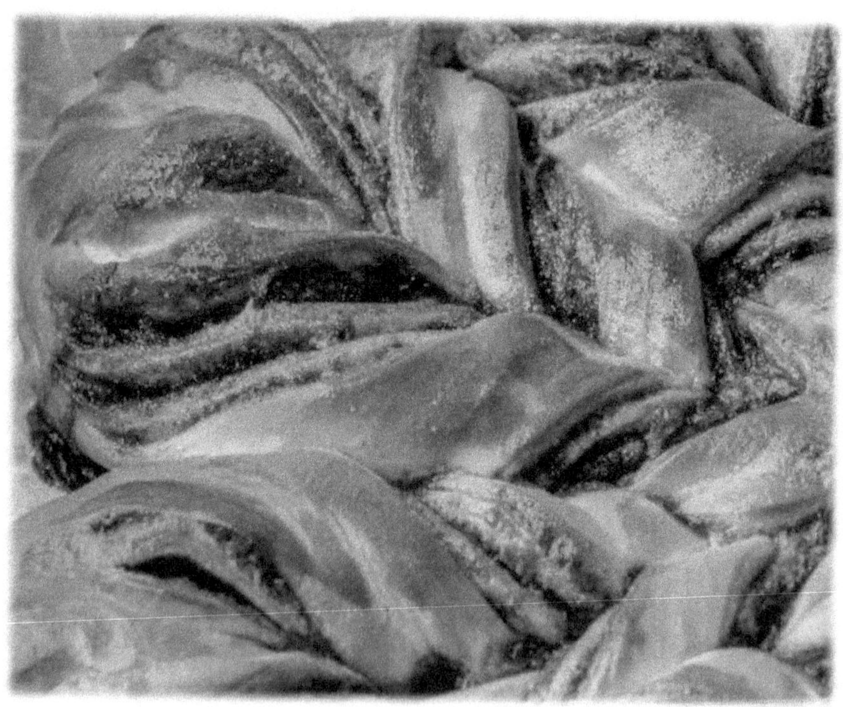

CHAPTER 10

Your Sourdough Q&A and Troubleshooting Guide

Greetings, fellow explorers of sourdough! We have mastered the art of fermentation and crafted our loaves into flawless golden shapes. However, the sourdough voyage may be an exciting one, let's face it. Fear not, brave bakers; this chapter guides you through the occasionally murky seas of baking mistakes, dietary modifications, and startup concerns. Get ready to respond to the urgent queries that keep you up at night (or perhaps you're simply lustfully gazing at your boiling starter).

Starter SOS: Calming Common Concerns

My starter isn't bubbling! Is it no longer alive? Calm down! A slow start is not always a sign of doom. Try a different flour, check the temperature (70–80°F is excellent!), and modify feeding schedules. Oh, young grasshopper, patience!

Hooch alert! Do I need to freak out? Be at ease! Just the excess byproducts of fermentation are responsible for this safe liquid separation. Just whisk it back in, add your starter, and continue.

My starter has an off-putting scent! Should I run? Not necessarily! A fragrance that is tart and yeasty is usual. However, it may be spoilt if it smells like gym socks or nail polish remover. Discard out everything and begin over.

Baking Blunders: From Dense Dough to Burnt Bottoms

My loaf is heavy and dense! What went amiss? Possible causes include over kneading, under fermenting, or using too much flour. Play with the amount of water in your dough, adjust your kneading technique, and let it rise completely.

My crust is completely burned! What happened? You may need to adjust the baking time or use a hot oven. To ensure uniform heat distribution, calibrate your oven's temperature, modify baking timings according to the size of your loaf, and think about utilizing a baking stone.

My bread feels sticky! Have I changed into a bear? There's nothing out of the ordinary about you! A sticky crumb might result from over fermenting or under baking. Be sure to modify the baking time and keep a close eye on the rising timings.

Ingredient Swaps and Dietary Delights:

Gluten-free flour? Can I still play? Of course! Examine gluten-free flour blends, such as rice or almond flours, and modify the amount of hydration as necessary. Keep in mind that while gluten-free sourdough may differ in texture, it can still taste great!

Dairy-free dreams? Come on, let's bake! Replace dairy milk with plant-based substitutes such as almond or oat milk. Your sourdough adventure may still be creamy and enjoyable, even if you have to make a small adjustment to your moisture levels.

Sugar blues? Be at ease! To make a healthy sourdough loaf, cut back on or completely remove additional sugars from your recipes. Try adding a little sweetness with natural sweeteners like dates or honey.

Bonus Tip: Keep a baking journal! Jot down your observations, notes, and recipes. Because it will assist you in monitoring your development, determining what works (and what doesn't!), and crafting your own masterpieces made with sourdough.

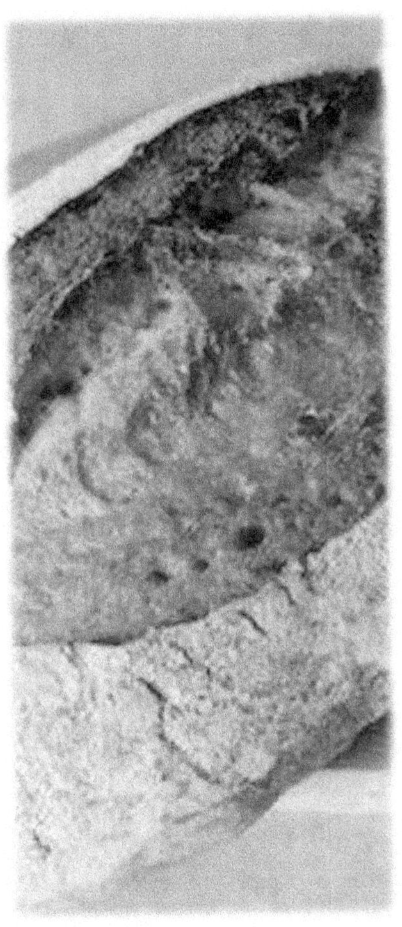 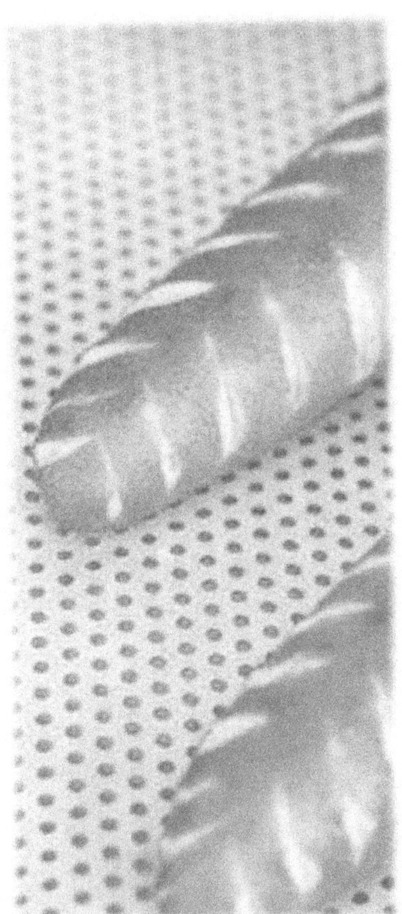

CONCLUSION

Bread lovers, this is the last rise—the point at which our sourdough journey without gluten culminates in a harmonious blend of delicious loaves and cherished memories. We have conquered the pinnacles of fermentation, fashioned gilded works of art from plain dough, and sailed through the occasionally murky seas of baking disasters and starter anxieties. Moreover, we've found that bread's soul-satisfying charm need not be lost when gluten is excluded.

Unlike any other book, this one has served as a testimony to the infinite possibilities of sourdough. We've discovered the secret depths of gluten-free flours, celebrated their distinctive dance, and created loaves that sing with every mouthful. We now know how to dance with our starters, fostering their acidic murmurs and witnessing their life burst forth. We've overcome the obstacles, rejoiced in the accomplishments, and come away with renewed admiration for the art of baking bread.

But the relationships made along the way are more important than the bread on this journey. We've commiserated over burned crusts and gooey crumbs, exchanged success stories, and urged one another to keep kneading, shaping, and baking. We've created a community where being gluten-free doesn't mean being alone; instead, it means sharing a love of bread and the excitement of making things.

As we finish this book, let the smell of freshly baked sourdough remain in our memories. Let it serve as a constant reminder of the many possibilities that may be created with only a bowl of flour, water, and a tiny bit of wild yeast. Let it serve as a monument to our grit, ingenuity, and undying devotion to warm, crusty bread.

It's not farewell, but rather a "see you soon." The quest for gluten-free sourdough is never-ending, including the continuous exploration of novel flours, textures, and tastes. Continue learning, experimenting, and baking with delight. Remember that the ideal loaf is always only one batch away, ready to be created by your own special sourdough magic.

With a smile as warm as a freshly baked loaf and a heart full of flour dust, I say goodbye to you. Adventurers, go forth and bake your way into a realm of magic that is gluten-free sourdough baking.

Like always, happy baking!